Multiple Choice Questions for Physiology

1. Which subject deals with the integrated functions of the body.
a. Histology   b. Anatomy   c. Physiology   d. Psychology
Correct answer (c)

2. Which functional groups are formed by the association of various tissues.
a. System   b. Body   c. Skeleton   d. Organ
Correct answer (d)

3. What is the thickness of cell membrane
a. 70-100°A   b. 100-150°A   c. 30-60°A   d. 10-20°A
Correct answer (a)

4. Cell physiology includes application of most of law's of which subjects.
a. Biology   b. Chemistry   c. Physics and Chemistry   d. Physics
Correct answer (c)

5. The properties of cell that are equated with those of life includes.
a. Growth   b. Reproduction   c. Metabolism   d. all
Correct answer (d)

6. Failure of a tissue or organ to develop is called.
a. Hypoplasia   b. Aplasia   c. Neoplasia   d. Alopecia
Correct answer (b)

7. Following processes can occur across the cell membrane at the same time.
a. Osmosis   b. Active transport   c. Both   d. None of them
Correct answer (c)

8. The process of taking dissolved material into the substance of the cell is called.
a. Phagocytosis   b. Pinocytosis   c. absorption   d. diffusion
Correct answer (c)

9. The process by which cell can take in fluid and molecules too large to be carried across the plasma membrane by active transport is called
a. phagocytosis   b. Pinocytosis   c. absorption   d. diffusion
Correct answer (b)

10. If useful products are released from the cell. The process is called
a. secretion   b. excretion   c. sweating   d. urination
Correct answer (a)

11. The property of being able to react to a stimulus is called.
a. conductivity   b. Irritability   c. contractility   d. transmission
Correct answer (b)

12. The property of transmitting an impulse from one point in the cell to another.
a. conductivity   b. Irritability   c. contractility   d. transmission
Correct answer (a)

13. The property of shortening of cell in one direction is called
a. conductivity   b. Irritability   c. contractility   d. transmission
Correct answer (c)

14. The largest constituent of protoplasm is
a. Proteins   b. water   c. lipids   d. Inorganics
Correct answer (b)

15. Water occurs in the cell as
a. free water   b. bound water   c. both   d. none of them
Correct answer (c)

16. How much percentage of water lies within the body cells.
a. 20%   b. 40%   c. 60%   d. 80%
Correct answer (b)

17. How much percentage of water lies between the cells.
a.. 5%   b. 10%   c. 15%   d. 20%
Correct answer (c)

18. How much percentage of the body water by weight is in the blood plasma.
a. 1%   b. 5%   c. 10%   d. 15%
Correct answer (b)

19. Metabolic water is the water generated in all cell of the body by
a. ribosome   b. mitochondria   c.   bodies   d. centrosome
Correct answer (b)

20. The second largest constituent of protoplasm is
a. water   b. proteins   c. lipids   d. Inorganics
Correct answer (b)

21. Some proteins serve as structural element in
a. hair   b. wool   c. horn   d. all of them
Correct answer (d)

22. Immunity depends on which constituent as antibiodies
a. carbohydrates   b. Proteins   c. lipid   d. fats
Correct answer (b)

23. Which protein represent about 30% of the total protein content of the animal body.
a. Collagens   b. Elastins   c. Keratins   d. Fibrin
Correct answer (a)

24. The proteins of wool, hair, horns etc. is called
a. Collagens   b. Elastins   c. Keratins   d. Fibrin
Correct answer (c)

25. Reactive proteins include
a. Enzymes   b. Hormones   c. Globulins of blood d. All
Correct answer (d)

26. Lipids includes
a. Triglycerides   b. waxes   c. Prostaglandins   d. All
Correct answer (d)

27. What percentage of the cell is made up of carbohydrates
a. 1%   b. 2%   c. 3%   d. 4%
Correct answer (a)

28. Energy can be stored more efficiently as
a. Carbohydrates   b. Fats   c. Proteins   d. Water
Correct answer (b)

29. Which constituent in the cell has a high rate of utilization as energy
a. Carbohydrates   b. Fats   c. Proteins   d. Water
Correct answer (a)

30. RNA is intimately associated with synthesis of which constituent of the cell.
a. Carbohydrates   b. Proteins   c. Lipids   d. Inorganics
Correct answer (b)

31. How much percentage of inorganic material is contained in bones.
a. 35%   b. 45%   c. 55%   d. 65%
Correct answer (d)

32. Which mineral is an essential part of thyroxin
a. Fe   b. Mg   c. Iodine   d. Na
Correct answer (c)

33. Which mineral is essential part of hemoglobin
a. Iron   b. Iodine   c. sodium   d. magnesium
Correct answer (a)

34. Electrolytes are especially essential to which cells.
a. nerve   b. muscle   c. both   d. none of them
Correct answer

35. Which is the must abundant major ion found in the cells.
a. K+   b. HPO4   c. Mg   d. Na
Correct answer (a)

36. Proteins can exist in the cell in the forms of
a. Colloidal particles   b. crystalloid   c. Both   d. none
Correct answer (a)

37. Which transmembrane movement involves carriers?
a. facilitated diffusion   b. active transport   c. both   d. none of them
Correct answer (c)

38. Sugars depend on which mechanism to enter the cell
a. facilitated diffusion b. active transport   c. both   d. none of them
Correct answer (a)

39. The speed of entry of glucose is greatly increased by
a. oxytocin   b. insulin   c. glucagons   d. thyroxin
Correct answer (b)

40. Hygrometer is used to measure the
a. Water content   b. protein contents   c. lipid contents   d. mineral contents
Correct answer (a)

41. What percent solution of NaCl is considered isotonic to mammalian RBCs.
a. 0.8%   b. 0.85%   c. 0.90%   d. 0.95%
Correct answer (b)

42. If a bathing fluid has a lower osmotic pressure than the cell, it is called
a. Isotonic   b. hypotonic   c. hypertonic   d. All
Correct answer (b)

43. If a bathing fluid has higher osmotic pressure than the cell it is called
a. Isotonic   b. hypotonic   c. hypertonic   d. all
Correct answer (c)

44. If a bathing fluid has the same osmotic pressure than the cell it called
a. Isotonic   b. Hypertonic   c. hypotonic   d. all
Correct answer (a)

45. Crenation of Red cell occur, in
a. Isotonic solution   b. hypertonic solution c. hypotonic solution d. all
Correct answer (b)

46. Swelling/bursting of red cell occurs in
a. Isotonic solution   b. hypotonic solution c. hypertonic solution d. all
Correct answer (b)

47. Number of grams of solute per liter of solution is called
a. Normal solution   b. Molar solution   c. Molal solution   d. simple solution
Correct answer (b)

48. Number of gram equivalents of solute per liter of solution is called
a. Normal solution   b. Molar solution   c. molal solution   d. simple solution
Correct answer(a)

49. Number of gram of solute per 1000 gm of solvent is called
a. Normal solution   b. Molar solution   c. molal solution   d. simple solution
Correct answer (c)

50. Loss of water from tissues is called
a. hypotension   b. dehydration   c. edema   d. none of them
Correct answer (b)

51. Which ion is found in greater concentration outside the cell
a. K   b. Na   c. Cl   d. HCO_3
Correct answer (b)

52. Which ion is found in greater concentration inside the cell
a. K   b. Na   c. Cl   d. HCO_3
Correct answer (a)

53. Rough endoplasmic reticulum is involved in the synthesis of
a. glycogen   b. protein   c. steroids   d. lipids
Correct answer (b)

54. Smooth endoplasmic reticulum is involved in the synthesis of
a. glycogen   b. lipids   c. steroids   d. all
Correct answer (d)

55. The small spherical organelles attached to rough endoplasmic reticulum are called
a. vesicles   b. vacuoles   c. ribosome   d. polysomes
Correct answer (c)

56. Ribosomes help to synthesize
a. carbohydrates   b. proteins   c. lipids   d. minerals
Correct answer (b)

57. Enzymes involved in krebs cycle are localized in
a. ribosomes   b. mitochondria   c. polysomes   d. golgi bodies
Correct answer (b)

58. ATP is generated in
a. ribosomes   b. polysomes   c. mitochondria   d. golgi bodies
Correct answer (c)a

59. The mammalian cell that are known not to contain lysosomes are
a. WBc   b. RBc   c. Platellet   d. none of them
Correct answer (b)

60. Lysosome enzymes can degrade
a. Proteins   b. Carbohydrates   c. nucleic acid d. all
Correct answer (d)

61. Lysosomas are abundant in
a. RBc   b. WBC   c. Platelet   d. all
Correct answer (b)

62. Oxidase enzymes responsible for producing H_2O_2 are present in
a. Mitochondria   b. Ribosomes   c. Peroxisomes   d. Polysomes
Correct answer (c)

63. Microfilaments may assist
a. in the movement of fibroblasts in heart   b. growth of axons
c. contraction of all muscle   d. all
Correct answer (d)

64. Centriole consists of how many paired filaments
a. 5   b. 7   c. 9   d. 11
Correct answer (d)

65. The life span of RBc is of
a. 80 days   b. 100 days   c. 120 days   d. 140 days
Correct answer (c)

66. Following nucleotides are called purines
a. adenine   b. guanine   c. both   d. none
Correct answer (c)

67. Following nuclestides are called pyrimidine

a. adenine   b. guanine   c. cytosine   d. all
Correct answer (c)

68. Pyrimidine thymine occurs only in
a. RNA   b. DNA   c. Both   d. All
Correct answer (b)

69. Pyrimidine uracil occurs only in
a. RNA   b. DNA   c. Both   d. None of them
Correct answer (a)

70. Adenine is always paired with
a. guanine   b. cytosine   c. thymine   d. uracil
Correct answer (c)

71. Guanine is always paired with
a. adenine   b. cytosine   c. thymine   d. uracil
Correct answer (b)

72. During starvation of cell, the amount of following may decrease
a. RNA   b. Protein   c. Both   d. None of them
Correct answer (c)

73. The period between active cell divisions in called
a. anaphase   b. metaphase   c. interphase   d. telephase
Correct answer (c)

74. The chromatids become visible in
a. interphase   b. prophase   c. anaphase   d. metaphase
Correct answer (b)

75. The period of cell division when the nuclear envelop and nucleolus totally disappear is called
a. Prophase   b. Metaphase   c. anaphase   d. telophase
Correct answer (b)

76. The stage in which each centromere divides is called
a. Prophase   b. Metaphase   c. anaphase   d. telophase
Correct answer (c)

77. The division of cytoplasm is called
a. Telophase   b. Metaphase   c. Cytokinesis   d. None of them
Correct answer (c)

78. The following cell division occurs during gametogenesis

a. Mitosis   b. Meiosis   c. Both   d. None of them
Correct answer (c)

79. Crossing over is followed by
a. Meiotic division I   b. Meiotic division II, c. Both   d. None
Correct answer (c)

80. Each new sex cell is called
a. Gamete   b. embryo   c. zygote   d. -----
Correct answer (a)

81. The following are germ layer origin of tissues
a. ectoderm   b. mesoderm   c. endoderm   d. All
Correct answer (d)

82. Ectoderm forms
a. Epidermis   b. Blood   c. larynx   d. All
Correct answer (a)

83. Mesoderm form
a. Muscles   b. Bone ---   c. gonad   d. All
Correct answer (d)

84. Endoderm forms
a. digestive tube   b. kidney   c. nails   muscles
Correct answer (a)

85. External stimuli includes
a. light   b. temperature   c. touch   d. all
Correct answer (d)

86. The fundamental structural and functional unit of nerves system is
a. axon   b. dendrite   c. cell body   d. neurons
Correct answer (d)

87. The protoplasm   b. cytoplasm   c. Both   d. none
Correct answer (a)

88. The resting potential in nerves is produced by difference in
a. ions   b. charges   c. both   d. none of them
Correct answer (c)

89. Positively charged ions are called
a. anions   b. cations   c. both   d. none of them
Correct answer (b)

90. Negatively charged ions are called
a. anions   b. cations   c. both   d. none of them
Correct answer (a)

91. In most nerve and muscle cell, the membrane potential is
a. 60 mv   b. 70 mv   c. 85 mv   d. 100 mv
Correct answer (c)

92. The plasma membrane in resting condition is almost impermeable to
a. K+   b. Na+   c. Cl   d. HCo3
Correct answer (b)

93. Plasma membrane in resting condition is very permeable to
a. K   b. Cl   c. Both   d. None of them
Correct answer

94. Which ion is actively transported to the outside of cell membrane
a. K   b. Cl   c. Na   d. HCo3
Correct answer (c)

95. Which ion moves freely through the plasma membrane
a. Na   b. Cl   c. k   d. HCo3
Correct answer (b)

96. The pumping of Na+ depends on
a. ADP   b. ATP   c. GDP   d. All
Correct answer (b)

97. The nerve fiber is capable of converting which stimuli to electrical energy
a. Mechanical   b. chemical   c. Both   d. none of them
Correct answer (c)

98. A nerve impulse is essentially a wave of
a. mechanical charge   b. electrical charge   c. Both   d. None
Correct answer (b)

99. Stimuli can be
a. electrical   b. mechanical   c. chemical   d. none
Correct answer (d)

100. In the living animal most stimuli are of
a. Physical nature   b. chemical nature   c. both   d. none
Correct answer (c)

101. Which process begins after Na influx essentially stops at its plateu
a. Depolarization   b. Repolarization   c. both   d. none
Correct answer (b)

102. The time when K+ is moving out of the cell is called
a. relative refractory period   b. absolute refractory period   c. both   d. none of them
Correct answer (a)

103. The following processes depend on changes in membrane conductance to Na and K.
a. Action potential   b. depolarization   c. repolarization   d. all of them
Correct answer (d)

104. Conductance is reciprocal of
a. permeability   b. action potential   c. resistance   d. depolarization
Correct answer (c)

105. Propagation of action potential is called
a. Repolarization   b. depolarization   c. nerve impulse   d. none of them
Correct answer (c)

106. Propagation in nerves normally proceed in
a. one direction   b. two direction   c. both   d. none of them
Correct answer (a)

107. Large diameter fibers propagate action potential at
a. lower velocities   b. higher velocities   c. equal velocities   d. none of them
Correct answer (b)

108. Presynaptic neurons conduct impulses
a. toward the synapse   b. away from the synapse   c. both correct   d. both in correct
Correct answer: (a)

109. Following morphine like substance are found in the thalamus of the brain
a. Enkephalins   b. endorphins   c. both   d. none of them
Correct answer (c)

110. Following are presumed to act as transmitters in the natural control of pain
a. Enkephalins   b. endorphins   c. both   d. none of them
Correct answer (c)

111. Following drugs act at the synapse level.
a. morphine   b. strychnine   c. tranquilizers   d. All
Correct answer (d)

112. Neuron excitability increase in
a. alkalosis   b. acidosis   c. neutral   d. none of them

Correct answer (a)

13. Neuron excitability decreases in
a. alkalosis   b. acidosis   c. neutral   d. none of them
Correct answer (b)

114. Neural excitability is not affected by
a. alkalosis   b. acidosis   c. neutral   d. none of them
Correct answer (d)

115. Inhibitory transmitters may be
a. glycine   b. GABA   c. both   d. none of them
Correct answer (c)

116. Action potential in nerve fibers differ in
a. magnitude   b. duration   c. both   d. none of them
Correct answer (c)

117. Reflex arc is made up of a chain of at least
a. two neuron   b. three neurons   c. four neurons   d. five neurons
Correct answer (a)

118. The simplest reflex is
a. spinal reflex   b. stretch reflex   c. knee jerk   d. none of them
Correct answer (a)

119. Reflex center are located
a. through out the neurons system   b. in cervical region only
c. thoracic region only   d. In lumber region only
Correct answer (a)

120. The medulla oblongata contains reflex centers for control of
a. heart action   b. respiration   c. vomiting   d. all of them
Correct answer (d)

121. The reflex center associated with locomotion are situated in
a. Cerebrum   b. cerebellum   c. mid brain   d. Pons
Correct answer (b)

122. The reflex center associated with temperature regulation are situated in
a. cerebrum   b. cerebellum   c. hypothalamus   d. Pons
Correct answer (c)

123. Reflex activity decrease under the influence of
a. anesthetic   b. barbiturates   c. catamine   d. all
Correct answer (d)

124. Reflexes associated with the animal nerves include
a. corneal reflex   b. papillary reflex   c. auditory reflex   d. all of them
Correct answer (d)

125. Homeostasis is controlled by regulating the activity of
a. cardiac muscle   b. smooth muscle   c. gland   d. all
Correct answer (d)

126. The major integrator of autonomic nervous system is
a. cerebrum   b. cerebellum   c. hypothalamus   d. all
Correct answer (c)

127. Each preganglionic axon braches and can therefore synapse, with as many as
a. 4 neurons   b. 6 neurons   c. 8 neurons   d. 10 neurons
Correct answer (d)

128. Most organ of the body receive innervations
a. sympathetic   b. parasympathetic   c. both   d. non
Correct answer (c)

129. Cell membranes
a. consist almost entirely of protein molecules
b. are impermeable to fat-soluble substances
c. in some tissues permit the transport of glucose at a greater rate in the presence of insulin
d. are freely permeable to electrolytes but not to proteins
e. have a stable composition throughout the life of the cell
Correct answer: ©

130. The primary force moving water molecules from the blood plasma to the interstitial fluid is
a. active transport
b. cotransport with H+
c. facilitated diffusion
d. cotransport with Na+
e. filtration
Correct answer: (E)

131. Second messengers
a. are substances that interact with first messengers inside cells
b. are substances that bind to first messengers in the cell membrane
c. are hormones secreted by cells in response to stimulation by another hormone
d. mediate the intracellular responses to many different hormonesand neurotransmitters
e. are not formed in the brain
Correct answer (d)

132. The resting membrane potential of a cell
a. is dependent on the permeability of the cell membrane to K+ being greater than the permeability to Na+
b. falls to zero immediately when Na+, K+ ATPase in the membrane is inhibited
c. is usually equal to the equilibrium potential for K+
d. is usually equal to the equilibrium potential for Na+
e. is markedly altered if the extracellular Na+ concentration is increased
Correct answer (a)

133. Proteins that are secreted by cells are generally
a. not synthesized on membrane-bound ribosomes
b. initially synthesized with a signal peptide or leader sequence at their C terminal
c. found in vesicles and secretory granules
d. moved across the cell membranes by endocytosis
e. secreted in a form that is larger than the form present in the endoplasmic reticulum
Correct answer (c)

134. Osmosis is
a. movement of solvent across a semipermeable membrane from an area where the hydrostatic pressure is high to an area where the hydrostatic pressure is low
b. movement of solute across a semipermeable membrane from an area in which it is in low concentration to an area in which it is in high concentration
c. movement of solute across a sempermeable membrane from an area in which it is in high concentration to an area in which it is in low concentration
d. movement of solvent across a semipermeable membrane from an area in which it is in low concentration to an area in which it is in high concentration
e. movement of solvent across a semipermeable membrane from an area in which it is in high concentration to an area in which it is in low concentration
Correct answer (e)

135. Deuterium oxide and inulin are injected into a normal 30-year-old man. The volume of distribution of deuterium oxide is found to be 42 L and that of inulin 14 L.
a. The man's intracellular fluid volume is about 14 L.
b. The man's intracellular fluid volume is about 28 L.
c. The man's plasma volume is about 7 L.
d. The man's interstitial fluid volume is about 9 L.
e. The man's total body water cannot be calculated from these data.
Correct answer (b)

136. Which of the following receptors does not span the cell membrane 7 times
a. β-Adrenergic receptor
b. Rhodopsin
c. 5-HTic receptor
d. Mineralocorticoid receptor
e. LH receptor
Correct answer (d)

137. Which of the following does not act interacellularly to produce physiologic effects
a. Triiodothyronine
b. Inositol triphosphate
c. Aldosterone
d. Cyclic AMP
e. Doapamine
Correct answer (e)

138. The action potential of a neuron
a. is initiated by efflux of Na+
b. is terminated by efflux of K+
c. declines in amplitude as it moves along the axon
d. results in a transient reversal of the concentration gradient of Na+ across the cell membrane
e. is not associated with any net movement of Na+ or K+ across the cell membrane
Correct answer (b)

139. A squid axon is placed on stimulating electrodes, and an intracellular electrode is inserted and connected through a cathode-ray oscilloscope (CRO) to an indifferent electrode. When the axon is stimulated, the latent period is 1.5 ms. The intracellular electrode is 6 cm form the anode of the simulator and 4.5 cm from the cathode of the simulator. What is the conduction velocity of the axon.
a. 15 m/s
b. 30 m/s
c. 40 m/s
d. 67.5 m/s
e. This cannot be determined from the information given.
Correct answer (b)

140 Which of the following has the slowest conduction velocity.
a. alpha fibers   b. beta fibers   c. gamma fibers   d. B fibers   e. C fibers
Correct answer (e)

141. Which part of the neuron has the highest concentration of Na.
a. dendrites   b. cell body   c. synaptic knobs   d. none of them
Correct answer (d)

142. Which of the following statements about nerve growth factor is not true
a. it is made up of 3 polypeptide subunits
b. it is found in high concentration in the submaxillary salivery gland
c. it is picked up by nerves from the organs they innervate
d. it is present in brain.
Correct answer (b)

143. The ciliary ganglion:
a. is found between the optic nerve and the medial rectus
b. contains sympathetic nerve that supplies the sphincter pupillae
c. is a parasympathetic relay ganglion for fibers from the Edinger-Westphal nucleus
d. contains sensory nerve
e. has a motor nerve that goes to the inferior oblique
Correct Answer: c,d

144. The nasociliary nerve supplies:
a. the sphenoidal sinus
b. ethmoidal sinus
c. cornea
d. lacrimal sac
e. all above
Correct Answer: e

145. The cornea:
a. is thicker centrally than peripherally
b. contains 10,000 endothelium cells per square mm at birth
c.has an acellular collagenous stroma
d. contain Descemet's membrane is produced by the endothelium
e. has a refractive index of 1.38
Correct Answer: d,e

146. The vitreous:
a. is firmly attached to the pars plana
b. has a high concentration of hyaluronic acid
c. contains calcium in asteroid hyalosis
d. all above
Correct answer: d

147. The globe:
a. is closer to the orbital floor than the roof
b. is closer to the lateral wall of the orbital cavity than to medial wall
c. has a vertical diameter less than the anteroposterior diameter
d. has an anterior segment which form 1/4 of the circumference
e is least protected laterally
Correct Answer: b,c

148. The following are true about lacrimal gland:
a. the palpebral part drains into the superior conjunctival fornix through 12 ducts
b. the palpebral part of the gland is 1/3 the size of the orbital part
c. excision of palpebral but no the orbital part abolish the tear secretion by the gland
d. it receives secretomotor nerve from the third cranial nerve

e. the lymphatic drainage is to parotid gland
 Correct Answer: a,b

149. With regard to the lacrimal drainage system:
a. the upper lacrimal punctum is lateral to the lower punctum
b. the lacrimal canaliculi are lined by stratified squamous epithelium
c. nasolacrimal duct is narrowest at the lowest end
d. nasolacrimal duct runs downwards, lateral and forwards to the anterior part of inferior meatus
e. congenital blockage is due mainly to delay development of common canaliculus
 Correct Answer: a,b

150. The cells of the retinal pigment epithelium:
a. are of mesenchymal origin
b. are shorter at the fovea than else where in the retina
c. have intracellular melanosomes
d. regenerate visual pigment
e. form the inner outer blood-retina barrier
 Correct Answer: c,d

151. The optic chiasm:
a. forms the floor of the recess of the third ventricle
b. is inferior to the medial root of the olfactory tract
c. has the internal carotid artery as its immediate lateral relation
d. all above
 Correct Answer; d

152. True statement about the facial nerve include:
a its nucleus is in the floor of the fourth ventricle
b. its fibres reach the surface of the brain in the cerebellopontine angle
c. transmits taste fibres for the anterior half of the tongue
d. all above
 Correct Answer; d

153. The following are true about cerebrospinal fluid:
a. it is found in the space between the pia mater and the arachnoid
b. the normal amount in human being is about 500 ml
c. with the body lying in lateral horizontal position, the normal intracranial pressure is about 100 ml of water
d. only the lateral ventricle contains choroidal plexus which secrete cerebrospinal fluid
e. cerebrospinal fluid contains the same concentration of glucose as the blood
 Correct Answer:a,c

154. The parotid gland:

a. contains a fascial sheath which is innervated by second cervical nerve
b. receives post-ganglionic parasympathetic nerve from the otic ganglion
c. contains a duct which opens into the mouth opposite the upper canine tooth
d. is composed of serous acini which contribute to the saliva
e. is covered by the massenter
Correct Answer; a, b, d

155. In the head and neck:
a. the lymph from the upper lid drains to the parotid and submandibular lymph nodes
b. the facial nerve comes from the first pharyngeal arch
c. branches of the ophthalmic division of the trigeminal nerve supply the skin of the scalp as far backward as the vertex
d. the veins of the scalp are connected to both the diploic veins and the intracranial venous sinuses
e. an unilateral cleft lip is a failure of the maxillary process to fuse with the medial nasal process
Correct Answer; c, d

156. In the development of the eye:
 a. the orbit is completed by 10th week of gestation
 b. the orbit arises from fusion between the lateral nasal process and the maxilla
 c. the lower eyelids are formed by the maxillary process
 d. all above
Correct Answer; d

157. The following structures are of ectodermal origin:

a. the retina and its retinal pigment epithelium
b. iris stroma
c. the sclera
d. the ciliary muscle
e. the corneal stroma
 Correct Answer; a,e

158. The hyaloid artery:
a. arises from the dorsal ophthalmic artery
b. communicates freely with the choroidal circulation throughout development
c. regresses after birth
d. Bergmeister's papillae is a remnant
e. forms part of the vascular propria lentis
 Correct Answer; a,d

159. With respect to lens development:
a. the lens first appears at 27 days of gestation
b. it is formed from neural crest cells
c. the lens first appears as a vesicles with a single layer of epithelial cells

d. Y suture is absent in the embryonic nucleus
e. the adult lens is more spherical than the foetal
 Correct Answer; a, c, d

160. The following structures arise from the first pharyngeal arch:
a. common carotid artery
b. mandible
c. facial nerve
d. orbicularis oculi
e. temporalis
Correct Answer; b,e

161. Glucagon:
a. is secreted by beta-islet cell of pancreas
b. is a polypeptide hormone
c. has a positive cardiac inotropic effect
d. causes gluconeogenesis in the liver
e. causes glycogenolysis in the liver
 Correct Answer; b, c, d

162. During accommodation for near:
a. the spherical aberration of the eye increases
b. the ciliary muscle relaxes
c. the field of vision decreases
d. the amount of light entering the eye increases
e. the thickness of the lens increases
Correct Answer; c, e

163. In binocular vision:
a. only points on the horopter fall on the corresponding retinal point
b. points in front of the horopter will stimulate binasal retina
c. points outside the horopter is perceived doubly
d. the Panum's fusional area is wider in the centre than the periphery
e. sensory fusion refers to the cortical integration of images perceived by the two eyes
 Correct Answer; a, e

164. The following are true about entopic phenomenon:
a. it can be produced by cells in the vitreous
b. it can be produced by palpation of the eyeballs
c. the size of one's pupil can be observed with a pinhole
d. asteroid hyalosis causes significant visual disturbance due to entopic phenomenon
e. Haidinger's brushes are produced by the inner plexiform layers
 Correct Answer; c, e

165. The retinal pigment epithelium cells:

a. esterify and store excess retinol

b. transport retinol binding protein from blood to subretinal space

c. are secured laterally to each other by tight junction

d. all above

Correct Answer; d

166. The intraocular pressure can fluctuate:

a. seasonally

b. diurnally

c. with eye movements

d. all above

Correct Answer; d

167. The tear film:

a. contributes to the refractive function of the eye

b. is partly formed from the goblet cells

c. is 100um thick

d. its normal break-up time is 5 to 15 seconds

e. is decreased with topical atropine

Correct Answer; a, b

168. The human lens:

a. has a higher refractive index in the nucleus than the cortex

b. contains a higher potassium concentration than the aqueous

c. contains a higher concentration of sorbitol in diabetic patient than normal population

d. all above

Correct Answer; d

169. True statement about dark adaptation include:

a. there is a shift in peak spectral sensitivity from 555 nm to 505 nm with dark adaptation

b. rods are more sensitive than cone during dark adaptation

c. biphasic changes only occur in retina which processes both rods and cones

d. all above

Correct Answer; d

170. During phototransduction:

a. hyperpolarisation occurs due to closure of the sodium channels

b. 11-cis-retinal molecules are converted to all-trans-retinal

c. transducin, a G protein converts GDP to GTP

d. all above

Correct Answer; d

171. With regard to the blood retina barrier:

a. the outer blood retina is formed by the retinal pigment epithelium cells and their junctions

b. the blood retina barrier is typically defective in the immediate perpapillary region

c. the retinal vascular endothelial cells can actively transport fluid and anions from the extracellular space of the retina into the circulation
d. all above
Correct Answer; d

172. True statements about the aqueous humour:
a. has a higher lactic acid concentration than in the plasma
b. the glucose levels is lower than that of the plasma levels
c. the ascorbic acid concentration is twice that of the plasma
d. it contains the same concentration of protein as in the plasma
e. the rate of formation is about 2.5ul/minute
 Correct Answer; a, e

173. Stretch reflex:
a. is a monosynaptic reflex with a response time of 1 msec
b. originates in the muscle spindle which sends off impulses in type Ia nerve fibres
c. is intensified by impulses in the gamma efferent fibres
d. all above
Correct Answer: d

174. Glycocylated haemoglobin:
a. is absent in the plasma of people without diabetes mellitus
b. results from the combination of a HbA and a sugar
c. when measured as HbA1c in plasma gives a more accurate retrospective estimates of blood sugar levels than other
    glycosylated products
d. all above
Correct answer: d

175. With regard to the autonomic nervous system:
a. the dorsal root ganglia is made up mainly of the cell bodies of the sympathetic nerves
b. the preganglionic sympathetic fibres are usually longer than preganglionic parasympathetic fibres
c. acetylcholine is the neurotransmitter at the ganglia of both sympathetic and parasympathetic nervous system
d. botulin toxin blocks acetylcholine receptors
 Correct Answer; a, c

176. The following are true about blood coagulation:
a. heparin inhibits blood coagulation through its interference with vitamin K metabolism in the liver
b. addition of vitamin K to freshly drawn blood delays clotting
c. thrombin converts fibrinogen to fibrin
d. platelets are essential for blood clot
 Correct Answer; c, d

177. In the inner ear:
a. endolymph is found in the tunnel of Corti
b. the lowest tone that be heard is 300 Hz
c. the perilymph has the same composition as the cerebrospinal fluid
d. the longer fibers of the basilar membrane are found at the apex
 Correct Answer; c, d

178. Regarding interferon:
a. it is a virus specific molecules
b. it acts by neutralizing exotoxin
c. it enhances the histocompatibility antigen on cell surface and thereby activate the T cells
d. it exerts its effect by integrating itself with the DNA of virus infected cells
 Correct Answer; c

179. Following an acute inflammation, the following may occur:
a. complete resolution
b. abscess formation
c. chronic inflammation
d. all above
Correct Answer: d

180. Acetazolamide causes the following:
a. metabolic acidosis
b. hyperkalaemia
c. hypernatraemia
d. renal calculi
e. hypercalcaemia
 Correct Answer: a, d

181. The effects of topically applied anticholinesterase on the eye include:
a. conjunctival hyperaemia
b. raised intraocular pressure
c. ciliary muscle contraction
d. sphincter pupillae muscle relaxation
e. retraction of the upper lids
 Correct Answer; c

182. Impaired accommodation occurs with:
a phenothiazine
b. topical pilocarpine
c. topical atropine
d. topical phenylephrine
Correct Answer; a, c

183. True statements about chloroquine include:

a. is safer than hydroxychloroquine at equivalent dose
b. can cause corneal deposition
c. causes posterior subcapsular cataract
d. chloroquine is bound to the melanin of the retinal pigment epithelium
e. causes reversible toxic maculopathy
 Correct Answer; b, d

184. At the adrenergic synapse, the concentration of adrenaline in synaptic cleft:
a. increased by cocaine which inhibit reuptake of adrenaline
b. decreased by MAO (monoamine oxidase) - inhibitors
c. controlled chiefly by the activity of the enzyme COMT
d. increased by noradrenaline receptor blockers
 Correct Answer; a, d

185. True statements about the nucleic acid include:
a. contains purine and pyrimidine which are bound together by covalent bonds
b. there is always an equal concentration of purine and pyrimidine
c. in RNA, thymine is replaced by uracil
d. introns is more common than exons on the DNA
e. the histones mark the excision site
 Correct Answer; b, c

186. In allergic reaction:
a. Arthus reaction is a type IV reaction
b. anaphylaxis occurs in patients who have had no previous exposure to the offending substance
c. contact dermatitis is a type IV reaction
d. positive Mantoux test is a type III reaction
 Correct Answer; c

187. With regard to immunoglobulin A:
a. it is the heaviest immunoglobulin
b. it is the first immunoglobulin to be produced when the body is invaded by viruses
c. it is secreted by the lacrimal gland
d. it is secreted in the breast milk
 Correct Answer; c, d

188. The following enzymes on the left are responsible for the synthesis of the neurotransmitters on the right:
a. monoamine oxidase: noradrenaline
b. cholinesterase: acetylcholine
c. catechol-o-methyl transferase: dopamine
d. dopa decarboxylase: adrenaline
Correct Answer; d

189. The following are true about the DNA in mitochondria:

a. they are found in the ovum and not the spermatozoan
b. they have their own genome
c. they are expressed in muscle cells
d. all above
Correct Answer: d

190. The following are true :
a. the HLA proteins are found within the cytoplasm of the cells
b. HLA class I antigens are expressed on all cells with nuclei
c. HLA class II antigens presents the virus infected cells to cytotoxic T lymphocytes
d. HLA genes are found on chromosome 6
e. HLA tissue typing is carried out in all forms of transplantation to prevent rejection
Correct Answer; b, d

191. True statements about chromosome include:
a. 23 chromosomes are found in germinal cells
b. in female only one chromosome is activated
c. the Barr body is due to inactivated X chromosome
e. all above
Correct Answer; d

192. Sodium fluorescein:

a. has a higher affinity for plasma protein than indocyanine green.

b. does not leak from the choroidal vasculature.

c. does not leak from normal retinal vasculature.

d. emits light of longer wavelengths than the one it
   absorbs.

Correct Anwer: c, d

193. Direct light reflex of the pupil is absent in:
a. lesion of the ipsilateral ciliary ganglion.

b. transaction of the ipsilateral optic nerve.

c. bilateral occipital lobe lesion.

d. topical application of phenylepherine.

Correct Anwer: a, b

194. The following conditions give rise to red blood cells with increased mean cell volume:
a. anaemia of chronic disease.

b. pernicious anaemia.

c. anaemia due to renal failure.

d. haemolytic anaemia.

Correct Anwer: b, d

195. Berry aneurysm:
a. is a congenital disorder.

b. is found most commonly in the posterior portion of the circle of Willis.

c. is symptomatic in majority of patients.

d. has absent intima elastica.

Correct Anwer: a, d

196. Regarding the human chromosomes:
a. there are 23 pairs autosomal chromosomes

b. the Y chromosome is larger than the X chromosome

c. cells containing YO chromosome are not compatible with life

d. Barr body is caused by the presence of an inactive X chromosome

Correct Answer: c, d

197. The following are true about erythromycin:
a. it can be used to treat chlamydial infection effectively

b. it decreases the renal excretion of cyclosporin

c. it causes cholestasis

d. all above

Correct Answer: d

198. In autosomal recessive inheritance:

a. the rarer the trait the higher the possibility of marriages within the same family

b. most recessive gene defects cause problem through failure to produce functional protein

c. both males and females are affected equally severely

d. all above

Correct Answer: d

199. The following structure arise from surface ectoderm:

a. conjunctival epithelium

b. lens

c. lacrimal gland

d. all above

Correct Answer: d

200. Lasers used in medicine include:

a. argon

b. carbon dioxide

c. helium

d. all above

Correct Answer: d

201. The following are true about tight junction:
a. it forms a barrier to water

b. it is found in the blood-aqueous barrier of the ciliary body

c. it is found in the blood-retinal barrier at the apex of the retinal pigment epithelium

d. all above

Correct Answer: d

202. The following are true about the dural venous sinuses:
a. they have no valve

b. the cavernous sinus is closely related to the pituitary gland

c. the cavernous sinus has the first two divisions of the trigeminal nerve on its lateral wall

d. all above

Correct Answer: d

203. True statements about the cerebral blood flow include:

a. it is constant for the blood pressure in the range between 50-150mmHg

b. hypocapnia causes vasoconstriction

c. cerebral arterioles constricts when the blood pressure raises

d. all above

Correct Answer: d

204. The following reflexes are used to test for brain stem death:
a. knee jerk reflex

b. Babinski's reflex

c. gag reflex

d. pupil reflex

Correct Answer: c, d

205. In injury of the peripheral nerve:
a. pure sensory or pure motor nerve tends to regenerate better than mixed nerve

b. in neuropraxia, there is anatomical disruption of the nerve

c. Wallerian degeneration occurs 3 days after the injury

d. Wallerian degeneration occurs proximal to the site of the injury

Correct Answer: a, c

206. The blood - brain barrier:

a. is permeable to bilirubin at birth

b. is formed by the tight junctions between endothlial cells and the end feet processes of astrocytes

c. is permeable to glucose

d. all above

Correct Answer: d

207. The following are true about DNA synthesis:
a. it requires DNA polymerase
b. reverse transcriptase enzymes are involved
c. moves in a 5'---> 3' direction
d. the rate of error in DNA synthesis is 1 in 10^5 base pairs
Correct Answer: a, c

208. With regard to DNA molecules:
a. they contain adenine, cytosine, guanine and uracil bases
b. they can be detected with Western blotting
c. they can be detected with Southern blotting
d. they are denatured at temperature of 100^0C
Correct Answer: c, d

209. G-proteins:
a. are activated by the binding of an extracellular ligand to a membrane receptor
b. can be mutated in tumour cells
c. mediate the action of glucocorticoid hormone
d. they are inactivated by cholera toxins.
Correct Answer: a, b

210. The following is true about gluconeogenesis:
a. it occurs in liver
b. it occurs in kidney
c. it occurs in adipose tissue
d. it is inhibited by glucagon
Correct Answer: a, b

211. With regard to membrane receptors for hormones:

a. they are often glycoproteins
b. they are important for hormones made up of steroid
c. those for insulin exhibit an intrinsic protein kinase activity
d. glucagon uses calcium as a second messenger

Correct Answer: a, c

212. With regard to interferons:
a. they are produced by B lymphocytes

b. IFN-gamma ☐is produced by cells infected with virus

c. IFN-gamma increases MCH class I and II expression in antigen presenting cell

d. IFN-gamma is produced by fibroblasts

Correct Answer: b, c

213. The following are true about interleukins 1 (IL-1):
a. it is produced mainly by the neutrophils

b. it stimulates the proliferation of B and T cells

c. it increases bone production

d. it acts on the hypothalamus to cause fever

Correct Answer: b, d

214. With regard to interleukins:

a. IL-2 is produced mainly by CD8+ cells

b. IL-3 stimulates the growth of haemopoietic stem cells

c. IL-4 increases the production of IL-1

d. IL-6 stimulates acute phase protein synthesis

Correct Answer: b, d

215. With regard to HLA class 1 antigen:

a. they are expressed on all nucleated cells

b. they are essential for viral antigen recognition by cytotoxic cells

c. the genes for HLA class 1 molecules are located on chromosome 6 and 15

d. all above

Correct Answer: d

216. The following are true about lymphocytes:

a. T cells account for 20% of the circulating lymphocytes

b. in the spleen, B cells are found in the periarteriolar areas of white pulp

c. in the lymph nodes, T cells occupy the paracortical area surrounding the germinal centres.

d. B cells but not T cells express surface Ig G

Correct Answer: c, d

217. In the complement system;
a. alternative pathway does not rely on antibody

b. C1 is the first enzyme complex in the classical pathway

c. both the alternative and classical pathway converge at C3

d. all above

Correct Answer: d

218. The following are true about the Fc regions of an immunoglobulins:

a. they can be cleaved from the Fab regions by papain

b. they are involved in mast cell binding

c. they are involved in the activation of the complement cascade

d. all above
Correct Answer: d

219. Type IV hypersensitivity responses:

a. typically occur 72 hours after contact with the antigen

b. occur in Kveim's test

c. occur in contact dermatitis

d. all above
Correct Answer: d

220. Ig G:
a. has a molecular weight of 150000

b. is the principal immunoglobulin in secondary immune response

c. is the most common circulating immunoglobulins in the serum

d. all above
Correct Answer: d

221. The following are true about antigen presenting cells (APC):
a. Langerhan's cells are the antigen presenting cells of the epidermis

b. CD8+ cells only recognize antigen presenting cells bearing MHC (major histocompatibility complex) class I

c. tumour necrosis factor alpha (TNF☐) can turn endothelial cells into antigen presenting cells

d. all above
Correct Answer: d

222. With regard to histones:
a. they are basic proteins

b. they are essential for the formation of stable DNA

c. mitochondria do not contain histones

d. all above
Correct Answer: d

223. In the regulation of genes:

a. more than 90% of the base sequences in human DNA have not known function

b. extrons are the part of the gene that code for amino acids found in the final proteins.

c. introns usually begins with the nucleotide sequence GT

d. all above
Correct Answer: d

224. Thromboxane A_2(TXA$_2$):
a. is derived from the membrane phospholipid

b. its production is decreased by non-steroidal anti-inflammatory drugs

c. causes platelet aggregation

d. all above
Correct Answer: d

225. In the lens:

a. the capsule is made up of type IV collagen

b. most metabolism is carried out in the anterior pole

c. hexokinase is a rate-limiting enzyme in carbohydrate metabolism

d. all above
Correct Answer: d

226. The following are true about the oxidation of glucose:

a. glycolysis produces 3% of the energy ultimately obtained from glucose

b. the first stage of glycolysis involves phosphorylation of glucose to
    1,6-fructose biphosphate.

c. glucose enters the Kreb's cycle as pyruvate

d. all above
Correct Answer: d

227. Amyloidosis:
a. the protein stained with Lugol's iodine

b. the deposition is extracellular

c. AL type is seen in 15% of patients with multiple myeloma.

d. all above
Correct Answer: d

228. Proto-oncogenes:

a. are only found in malignant tissues

b. are retroviruses capable of causing tumours

c. inactivates oncogenes

d. regulates cell growth and differentiation

Correct Answer: d

229. The following are true about G proteins:
a. they are first messengers

b. when activated, the alpha subunit exchange GDP for GTP

c. they are transmembrane signal receptor molecules

d. vibrio cholerae secrets an exotoxin which makes G-proteins resistant to inactivation

Correct Answer: b, d

230. True statements about p53 include:

a. a protein coded by a tumour suppressor gene

b. it suppresses mitosis

c. it is important regulators of apoptosis

d. all above
Correct Answer: d

231. Gout:
a. is characterized by hyperuricaemia.

b. causes scleritis

c. patient with gout should avoid eating offal

d. all above
Correct Answer: d

232. The following are true about cell-mediated immunity:
a. antigen-specific function is the role of the T-lymphocytes

b. cell-mediated immunity can activate the complement system

c. it is responsible for the delayed hypersensitivity reaction.

d. Gamma □interferon is an important mediator of B-cell activation.

Correct Answer: b

233. The following are useful in the diagnosis of HIV infection:

a. polymerase chain reaction

b. antibodies by enzyme-liked immunoadsorbent assay

c. P24 protein assay

d. all above

Correct Answer: d

234. The following are true about chemicals involved in allergic reaction:

a. thromboxane -leukocyte activation

b. prostaglandin-2 - vasodilatation

c. platelet-activating factor - leukocyte activation

d. heparin - augments inactivation of prostaglandins

Correct Answer: b

235. In AIDS, the following abnormalities are seen:

a. persistent lymphopenia

b. decreased interleukin-2 production

c. impaired delayed cutaneous hypersensitivity reactions

d. all above

Correct Answer: d

236. The following are true:

a. Ig G crosses the placenta

b. thymus gland is responsible for cellular immunity

c. C1-9 is used by the alternative complement pathway

d. eosinophils are responsible for phagocytosis

Correct Answer: a, b

237. Purines:
a. include guanine

b. are metabolized to uric acid

c. are mainly synthesized in the liver

d. all above

Correct Answer: d

238. Vitamin B12:

a. is essential for the metabolism of folic acid in
   the humans

b. is attached to a glycoprotein in the circulation

c. its deficiency is characterized by hypersegmentation of the neutrophils

d. all above

Correct Answer: d

239. Folic acid:

a. is water soluble

b. is absorbed in the stomach

c. deficiency leads to aplastic anaemia

d. deficiency occurs with methatrexate treatment

Correct Answer: a

240. Prostaglandins:

a. contains 20 carbon atoms

b. are unsaturated fatty acids containing a cyclopentane ring

c. the different types of prostaglandins are classified according to the configuration of the cyclopentane ring

d. all above

Correct Answer: d

241. The effect of sympathetic nervous system include:
a. contraction of the bladder detrusor muscle

b pupillary dilatation

c. reduced gastrointestinal motility

d. constricts bronchiole smooth muscle

Answer: b, c

242. The following are true about the smooth muscle cells:
a. presence of a striated appearance

b. do not contain actin and myosin

c. spontaneous muscle contraction

d. mitochondria are absent

Answer: c

243. The pain sensation
  a. arises from stimulation of free nerve endings

b. is transmitted to the central nervous system by
    unmyelinated C fibres

c. is transmitted to the brain via the spinothalamic tracts

d. is reduced by local anaesthetics through reduction of the
    potassium influx into the nerve fibres

Answer: a, b, c

244. The prothrombin time

a. assess the extrinsic pathway of the blood coagulation
   cascade

b. is prolonged in patients with fat absorption

c. is increased by warfarin

d. is increased by heparin

Answer: a, b, c

245. In human being, haemorrhage causes
a. venous constriction

b. decreased blood flow to the skin

c. a fall in cardiac output

d. splenic contraction

Answer: a, b, c

246. The light reflex involves the following structures:

a. Edinger-Westphal nucleus

b. ciliary ganglion

c. lateral geniculate body

d. oculomotor nerve

Answer: a, b,

247. The following are true about the autonomic nervous system:

a. the postganglionic neurones are largely unmyelinated

b. all preganglionic neurones are cholinergic

c. the preganglionic neurones of the sympathetic nervous system are
   shorter than the parasympathetic nervous system

d. the parasympathetic outflow is only found in the cranial nerves

Answer: a, b,c

248. The effects of glucocorticoid hormones include:
a. increase hepatic glycogen synthesis

b. decrease glucose uptake by the adipose tissue

c. decrease hepatic gluconeogesis

d. increase protein synthesis in the skeletal muscles

Answer: a, b

249. The secretion of insulin is stimulated by:
a. adrenaline

b. somatostatin

c. fatty acids

d. acetylcholine

Answer: c, d

250: Insulin:

a. is secreted as a pro-insulin

b. increases protein synthesis

c. is required for glucose uptake in all tissues

d. is a steroid hormone

Answer: a, b

251. The followings are steroid hormones:

a. corticotrophic hormone (ACTH)

b. aldosterone

c. thyroxine

d. growth hormone

Answer: b

252. The following have a lower concentration in the cerebrospinal fluid (CSF) than
plasma:

a. glucose

b. sodium

c. potassium

d. magnesium

Answer: d

253. The cerebrospinal fluid:

a. has a normal volume of 150 ml

b. has a normal opening pressure of 7 - 18 cm H_2O

c. flows from the ventricles to the subarachnoid space via the
foramen of Monro

d. does not contain neutrophils in normal individuals

Answer: a,b

254. The following sensations are conveyed in the dorsal column of the spinal cord:

a. pain

b. temperature

c. vibration

d. proprioception

Answer: c, d

255. In the neurones:

a. the axons convey impulse away from the cell body

b. neurotransmitters are synthesized in the cell bodies and then transported to the axons

c. the condition velocity increases with fibre diameter

d. the excitability is increased if the extracellular calcium concentration is decreased

Answer: a, c

256. Acetylcholine is a neurotransmitter at:

a. sweat glands

b. the adrenal medulla

c. parasympathetic ganglia

d. all above

Answer: d

257. Capillary permeability is increased by:

a. bradykinin

b. adrenaline

c. calcium

d. vasopressin

Answer: a

258. Glucagon:

a. is a positive inotrope

b. is produced by the beta cells of the pancreas

c. stimulates production of free fatty acids in the blood

d. its release is increased in starvation

Answer: a,c,d

259. Adrenaline:

        a. is synthesized by demethylation of noradrenaline

        b. increases coronary blood flow

        c. increases free fatty acids in the blood

        d. mobilizes glycogen stores from the liver

Answer: b,c,d

260. With reference to the skeletal muscle myofilaments

        a. actin is the major constituent of thin filaments

        b. myosin and tropomyosin combine to form the thick filaments

        c. troponin is a constituents of thin filaments

        d. tropomyosin prevents the interaction of actin and myosin in the resting state

Answer: a,c,d

261. Ablation of the stellate ganglion cuases:

        a. dilatation of the ipsilateral pupil

        b. vasodilatation of the ipsilateral arm

        c. posteral hypotension

        d. loss of consensual light reflex

Answer: b

262. Compared with intracellular fluid, extracellular fluid has,

        a. a greater osmolarity

        b. a higher protein concentration

        c. a lower chloride ion concentration

        d. a lower hydrogen ion concentration

Answer: d

263. The sequence of events in muscle contraction

        a. action potential depolarise the T-tubules

        b. depolarisation of T-tubules release calcium from sarcoplasmic reticulum

        c. calcium binds to the troponin-tropomycin complex

        d. all above

Answer: d

264. C fibres transmitting pain sensation

        a. are present in less numbers than A□ fibres in sensory nerves

        b. conduct at an average velocity of 2 metres/secon

        c. convey temperature sensation

        d. terminate in laminae 2 and 3 of the dorsal horn

Answer: c, d

265. A highly ionised drug:

        a. is well absorbed from the intestine

        b. is excreted mainly in the kidney

        c. crosses the placental barrier easily

        d. is reabsorbed from the renal tubule

Answer: a

266. The endothelium:

a. maintains the integrity of the corneal stroma through an
   ATP-Na+, K+-dependent pump

b. receives its nutrient from the blood vessels surrounding the cornea

c. undergoes multiplication in response to trauma

d. contains tight junction between adjacent endothelium

Answer: a,d

267. The following are true about the lens:

a. 90% of the weight of the lens is contributed by water.

b. it has no sensory innervation

c. the capsule is thicker posterior than anteriorly

d. it has an equatorial diameter of about 15 mm

Answer: b

268. Rod:
a. contains a cilium with a "9+0" configuration.

b. contains 11-trans-retinaldehyde essential for the absorption of photons

c. sheds its outer segment during the day

d. depolarize in response to flashes of light

Answer: a, c

269. The tear film:
a. has a higher pH than the serum

b. has a lower concentration of glucose than the serum

c. the oily component is secreted by the meibomian glands

d. all above

Answer: d

270. The following are water insoluble lens proteins:

a.☐ alpha crystalline

b. beta crystalline

c. gamma crystalline

d. all above

Answer: d

271. The retinal pigment epithelium (RPE):
a. is sensitive to hypervitaminosis A

b. isomerizes all-trans-retinal to 11-cis-retinol

c. does not undergo mitosis in response to injury

d. secrets the outer layer of the basal lamina that forms the Bruch's membrane.

Answer: b

272. The following are found in higher concentration in the tear than in the serum:
a. sodium

b. potassium

c. Ig G

d. glucose

Answer: b

273. The corneal stroma:
a. measures 500 um thick

b. transmits 90% of the incoming light

c. derives most of its oxygen from the precorneal tear film

d. is acellular which accounts for its transparency

Answer: a

274. The following proteins found in the tear of a normal person have antibacterial activity:

a. lysozyme

b. lymphokines

c. betalysin

d. immunoglobulin M

Answer: a,c

275. The following are true about electro-retinography?

a. flicker ERG can be used to test cone function

b. ERG is normal in patient with macular degeneration

c. the a-wave of ERG is produced by the ganglion cells

d. the b-wave is produced by the photoreceptor cells

Answer: a,b

276. Red blood cells:
a. measured 15 um in diameter

b. do not contain mitochondria

c. have a life span of 120 days in the circulation

d. are released from the bone marrow as mature erythrocytes

Answer: b, c

277. The following are true about the ABO and rhesus (Rh) system:
a. a person of group O is a universal donor

b. a person who is group AB has anti-A and anti-B antibodies

c. the presence of the D antigen means that the subject is Rh positive

d. rhesus antibodies occur naturally

Answer: a, c

278. The oxygen dissociation curve is shifted to the right with:

a. polycythaemia

b. pyrexia

c. respiratory acidosis

d. sickle cell anaemia

Answer: b, c,d

279. The intracranial pressure is decreased by:
a. intravenous mannitol

b. placing the patient in a head-up position

c. hyperventilation

d. all above
Answer: d

280. Dilatation of the peripheral arterial blood vessels can be caused by:
a. thromboxane A_2

b. adenosine diphosphate

c. endothelin

d. prostaglandins

Answer: d

281. The following signs occur in ipsilateral interruption of the cervical sympathetic trunk:

a. enophthalmos

b. ptosis

c. vasodilatation in the skin of the face

d.All above

Answer: d

282. The hypothalamus contains cells which are sensitive to:

a. PO_2

b. arterial blood pressure

c. [H+]

d. TSH (thyroid-stimulating hormone) concentration

Answer: d

283. The axons of the Purkinje cells in the cerebellar cortex:

a. terminate in excitatory synapses

b. terminate in cerebellar nuclei

c. terminate in the spinal cord.

d. form the main efferent pathway from the cerebellar cortex

Answer: b, d

284. The joint position sense of the right leg is impaired in damage of:

a. the superior colliculi

b. the cerebellum

c. the thalamus of the right

d. the post-central gyrus of the left cerebral hemisphere

Answer: d

285. The lateral spinothalamic tract:

a. carries fibres which terminate in the thalamus

b. contains mainly the second-order neurones.

c. carries fibres that carry information on temperature and pain

d. all above

Answer: d

286. In iron deficiency anaemia, the following is decreased:

a. MCV (mean cell volume)

b. ferritin

c. MCH (mean cell haemoglobin)

d. all above

Answer: d

287. The following are true about parathyroid hormone :
  a. it is an 84 amino acid peptide hormone

b. it increases calcium absorption from the gastrointestinal tract

c. it acts on a cell surface receptor that increases intracellular cyclic AMP

d. all above

Answer: d

288. Anti-diuretic diuretic hormone (ADH)
a. is synthesized by the posterior lobe of the pituitary gland

b. is released by neurosecretion

c. its secretion is increased by a low plasma osmolarity

d. increases the permeability of the distal convoluted tubule

Answer: b

289. The following are true about the thyroid hormone
a. iodide ions enter the follicle cells by passive diffusion

b .T4 and T3 bind to the receptors in nuclei

c. thyroxine, once synthesized, is coupled to thyroglobulin until released

d. a greater proportion of tri-iodothyronine is formed when iodine is deficient

Answer: b, c

290. True statements about aldosterone include:
a. it increases the amount of Na+-K+ ATPase in the target cells

b. it reduces the sodium content of the sweat

c. it increases the acidity of urine

d. all above

Answer: d

291. The following are true about the lens:
a. the anterior capsule is 10 times thicker than the posterior capsule

b. the anterior surface has a greater radius of curvature than the posterior surface

c. during accommodation the lens moves towards the cornea

d. the lens is more effective in absorbing light with long than short wave-lengths

Answer: b, c

292. The following are known to cause cataract:
a. prozac

b. simvastatin

c. salicylic acid

d. chlorpromazine

Answer: b, d

293. The following are associated with cataract formation:
a. dehydration

b. smoking

c. alcohol

d. all above

Answer: d

294. In the lens:
a. the potassium concentration is higher than that of the sodium

b. the majority of the lens protein are water soluble

c. glutathione is increased in the presence of cataract

d. all above

Answer: d

295. The following are true about crystallins found in the lens:
a. they are water soluble

b. alpha crystallin is the most common

c. gamma crystallin is the smallest crystallin

d. beta crystallin has the largest mass

Answer: a,c

296. With regard to the cornea:
a. photokeratitis occurs with wavelength of 270nm

b. microvilli are found in the outer layer of the epithelium

c. the turnover of the corneal epithelium typically takes 30 days

d. the corneal epithelium is about 10 layers in thickness

Answer: a,b

297. True statements about the aqueous include:

a. the production is about 2 ul/min

b. the endothelium contribute to the production of aqueous

c. its production decreases with age

d. all above

Answer: d

298. The following conditions can affect the pupil size:

a. iris colour

b. fatigue

c. exercise

d. all above

Answer: d

299. In Argyll-Robertson's pupils:

a. the pupils are irregular

b. iris atrophy are common

c. there are absent tendon reflexes

d. the lesion is in the mid-brain

Answer: a,b,c,d

300. The following are true about the pupils:

a. pupil size is largest in adolescence

b. physiological anisocoria is found in 20% of the population

c. the latent period of the pupil reaction to light ranges from 0.2 to 0.5s

d. all above

Answer: d

301. The effect of sympathetic nervous system include:
a. contraction of the bladder detrusor muscle

b pupillary dilatation

c. reduced gastrointestinal motility

d. constricts bronchiole smooth muscle

Answer: b, c

302. The following are true about the smooth muscle cells:
a. presence of a striated appearance

b. do not contain actin and myosin

c. spontaneous muscle contraction

d. mitochondria are absent

Answer: c

303. The pain sensation
   a. arises from stimulation of free nerve endings

b. is transmitted to the central nervous system by unmyelinated C fibres

c. is transmitted to the brain via the spinothalamic tracts

d. all above

Answer: d

304. The prothrombin time

a. assess the extrinsic pathway of the blood coagulation cascade

b. is prolonged in patients with fat absorption

c. is increased by warfarin

d. all above

Answer: d

305. In human being, haemorrhage causes
a. venous constriction

b. decreased blood flow to the skin

c. a fall in cardiac output

d. all above

Answer: d

306. The following are true about acetylcholine:
a. it is synthesized from acetyl-coenzyme A and choline

b. its formation is catalysed by acetylcholinesterase

c. at the synaptic cleft, it is inactivated by hydrolysis

d. reuptake by the presynaptic neurones play an important in inactivating acetylcholine

Answer: a, c

307. The following are true about acetylcholine receptors:
a. receptors at all autonomic ganglia are nicotinic

b. receptors at the skeletal neuromuscular junction are muscarinic

c. acetylcholine receptors in the autonomic ganglia can be selectively blocked by atropine

d. acetylcholine receptors in the neuromuscular junction can be selectively blocked by tubocurarine

Answer: a, d

308. The following are true about the muscarinic receptors:

a. they are found at the postganglionic parasympathetic synapses

b. they can be selectively blocked by atropine

c. M1 muscarinic receptors are found in the brain

d. all above

Answer: d

309. The following are true about the autonomic nervous system:
a. the preganglionic fibres are mainly myelinated, slow conducting B fibres

b. the postganglionic fibres are mainly unmyelinated C fibres

c. all preganglionic neurones are cholinergic neurons

d. all above

Answer: d

310. True statements about the following neurotransmitters include:

a. dopamine is formed from tyrosine

b. in the synapse, noradrenaline is inactivated by active reuptake into the presynpatic terminals

c. noradrenaline is formed by hydroxylation of dopamine

d. all above

Answer: d

311. The following are true about the tear film:
a. the normal volume is about 20 ul

b. its main protein content is made up of immunoglobulins

c. the lysozyme concentration is the greatest

d. the concentration of Ig A is greater than that of Ig G

Answer: c, d

312. With regard to the vitreous:
a. its water content is about 90%

b. its volume is about 5ml in each eye

c. its viscosity increases with age

d. its viscosity is contributed by the presence of sodium hyaluronate

Answer: d

313. True statements about saccadic eye movements include:
a. only occur when the patient is awake

b. the velocity is under voluntary control

c. the maximum velocity is 700 degrees / second

d. it has a latency of 250msec

Answer: c, d

314. The following are true about electroretinogram:
a. the a-wave is produced by the photoreceptors

b. the b-wave is produced by the ganglion cells

c. c-wave is produced by the retinal pigment epithelium

d. different light frequencies can be used to separate rod and cone response

Answer: a, c, d

315. The following are true:

a. the ratio of rod to cone is about 20:1

b. there are more ganglion cells in the retina than photoreceptors

c. the rod density is the highest nasal to the optic disc

d. the retinal artery is the main supply of nutrients to the photoreceptors

Answer: a

316. The following are true about the dural venous sinuses:
a. they have no valve

b. the cavernous sinus is closely related to the pituitary gland

c. the cavernous sinus has the first two divisions of the trigeminal nerve on its lateral wall

d. all above

Answer: d

317. True statements about the cerebral blood flow include:

a. it is constant for the blood pressure in the range between 50-150mmHg

b. the blood pressure is affected more by the PaO_2 than $PaCO_2$

c. hypocapnia causes vasoconstriction

d. cerebral arterioles constricts when the blood pressure raises

Answer: a, c, d

318. The following reflexes are used to test for brain stem death:
a. knee jerk reflex

b. Babinski's reflex

c. gag reflex

d. pupil reflex

Answer: c, d

319. In injury of the peripheral nerve:
a. pure sensory or pure motor nerve tends to regenerate better than mixed nerve

b. in neuropraxia, there is anatomical disruption of the nerve

c. Wallerian degeneration occurs 3 days after the injury

d. Wallerian degeneration occurs proximal to the site of the injury

Answer: a, c

320. The blood - brain barrier:
a. is permeable to bilirubin at birth

b. is formed by the tight junctions between endothlial cells and the end feet processes of astrocytes

c. is permeable to glucose

d. all above

Answer: d

321. The following are true about pain:
a. in disseminated cancer can be effectively relieved by hypophysectomy

b. does not ascend through the dorsal column of the spinal cord

c. is transmitted faster through the C fibres than the A delta fibres

d. stimulation of the ß receptors in the brain produces analgesia

Answer: a, d

322. The following are true about the spinal cord:

a. segment T12 lies at the level of vertebral body T9

b. cerebrospinal fluid is found within the subdural space

c. two point discrimination is transmitted in the dorsal column

d. hemisection results in contralateral loss of pain and temperature sense below the lesion.

Answer: a, c, d

323. Stimulation of the cholinergic pathway results in:

a. ciliary muscle contraction

b. a decrease in atrial contractility

c. gall bladder contraction

d. all above

Answer: d

324. The following drugs are miotics:
a. carbachol

b. cocaine

c. scopolamine

d. isofluorosphosphate

Answer: a, d

325. The following are true about the synaptic potential:

a. the Na^+ and K^+ currents occurs simultaneously

b. is a graded potential

c. the channel is ligand-gated

d. the post-synaptic potential is inhibitory when depolarizing

Answer: a, b, c

326. Cerebral blood flow is increase in:
a. chronic anaemia

b. inhalation of 5% carbon dioxide

c. seizures

d. inhalation of hyperbaric oxygen

Answer: a, b, c

327. The following are true about the sodium channels:

a. they are made up of polypeptide chains

b. have the highest densities at the nodes of Ranvier

c. open in response to depolarization

d. remain open as long as depolarization is maintained

Answer: a, b, c

328. The cerebral blood flow:
a. is increased by hypercapnia

b. is increased by hypoxia

c. accounts for 15% of the total cardiac output

d. all above

Answer: d

329. The blood-brain-barrier:

a. contains the foot processes of astrocytes

b. contains endothelial cells with tight junction

c. allows transport in one direction only ie from the vascular system into the brain

d. does not allow diffusion of water

Answer: a, d

330. The following are true about the antidiuretic hormone:
a. it is produced by the anterior pituitary gland

b. it reduces the cardiac output

c. it increases the renal absorption of sodium

d. it decreases the release of ACTH

Answer: b, c

331. The Pulfrich phenomenon:
a. occurs in patients with bilateral macular degeneration

b. occurs in optic neuritis

c. refers to the perception of photopsia

d. refers to the illusion of abnormal motion

Answer: b, d

332. The following are true about the contrast sensitivity:

a. Pelli-Robson chart tests the contrast sensitivity

b. is a measure of the ratio of brightness to darkness

c. a contrast of 1 means that there is no contrast

d. is highest at middle range frequencies

Answer: a, b, d

333. The following are true:
a. depth of perception only occurs in patients with normal visual acuities in both eye

b. Hering's law states that increased innervation to an extraocular muscle is accompanied by a decrease in innervation to its antagonists.

c. objects on the Panum's area fall on simultaneous areas of the retina

d. objects outside of the Panum's area are perceived as double

Answer: d

334. The following are yoke muscles:

a. right medial rectus and left lateral rectus

b. right inferior rectus and left superior rectus

c. right superior rectus and left inferior oblique

d. right superior oblique and left inferior rectus

Answer: a, c, d

335. The following are true about fluorescein sodium:

a. it is 60% bound to the plasma protein

b. it leaks out of the choriocapillaris readily

c. is excreted mainly by the kidney

d. it is excited by green light

Answer: b, c

336. When light fell on the eye, the pupil:
a. does not constrict if the optic nerve is severed

b. does not respond if the sympathetic system is not functioning

c. does not respond if the cholinergic system is blocked

d. does not respond if the pretectal nucleus is damaged

Answer: a, c, d

337. Rhodopsin:

a. is a red pigment

b. is least sensitive to red light

c. is regenerated when the eyes are closed

d. all above

Answer: d

338. The following are true about dark adaptation:
a. only regeneration of rhodopsin is responsible

b. adaptation usually takes about 20 minutes

c. dilatation of pupil plays a part in dark adaptation

d. it is better with the fovea than the peripheral retina

Answer: b,c

339. True statement about dark adaptation include:

a. the threshold for light intensity falls

b. it is biphasic

c. the initial adaptation is due to rod adaptation

d. the change in the light intensity threshold is usually around 100 folds

Answer: a, b,

340. Entoptic imagery may be caused by:

a.. opacities of the cornea

b. cells in the tear film

c. cells in the aqueous

d. vitreous cells

Answer: c, d

341. In the skeletal muscle:
a. myosin is found in the thick filament

b. the thin filament contains actin and troponin

c. during stimulus excitation calcium ions are derived from the serum

d. tropomyosin masks the myosin-combining sites on the actin

Answer: a, b, d

342. The conduction velocity of the nerve fibres is increased by:

a. decreased temperature

b. increased concentration of the external sodium ions

e. increased axon diameter

d. myelination

Answer: b, c, d

343. In the neurone:

a. the magnitude of the action potential is dependent on the strength of the stimulus

b. impulses can travel in both direction

c. depolarization is accompanied by increased permeability of the cell membrane to potassium ions

d. during depolarization, the potential of the neurone changes from -70mV to +40mV

Answer: b, c, d

344. The following are true about the neurotransmitters:

a. acetylcholine is inactivated mainly by presynaptic reuptake

b. tyrosine is essential for the formation of dopamine

c. noradrenaline is inactivated mainly by hydrolysis

d. adrenaline is formed from methylation of the noradrenaline

Answer: b, d

345. The muscle spindles:

a. are extrafusal fibres

b. are innervated by type Ia and II fibres

c. received motor innervation from the gamma fibres.

d. respond to tension in the muscle

Answer: b, c

346. During accommodation:
a. the distance between the lens and the ciliary body is decreased

b. the tension in the suspensory ligament is increased
c. the tension of the lens capsule is increased
d. the refractive power of the lens is increased

Answer: a, d

347. True statements about accommodation:

a. it does not occur in the absence of convergence
b. it occurs equally in both eyes
c. the range of accommodation decreases with age
d. the amplitude of accommodation is about 30D at birth

Answer: b,c

348. The visual acuity is affected by:

a. pupil size
b. illumination of the target
c. red-green colour blindness
d. contrast

Answer: a, b, d

349. The following are true about pupillary reaction to light:

a. it is impaired in damage of the Edinger-Westphal
   nucleus
b. it is impaired in damage of the ciliary ganglion
c. it is impaired in damage of the superior cervical ganglion
d. the pupil does not respond to light with a frequency of greater than 5 Hz

Answer: a, b, d

350. The following are true:

a. heroin causes miosis by increasing the release of acetylcholine.
b. botulinum toxin causes mydriasis by inhibiting the release of acetylcholine
c. phenylephrine causes mydriasis by stimulating the alpha ☐receptors
d. amphetamine causes mydriasis by inhibiting noradrenaline reuptake

Answer: b, c

351. The vitreous gel:
a. contains 98% water
b. is made up of 0.1% hyaluronic acid

c. is acellular

d. contains mainly type II and type III collagen

Answer: a

352. The following are true about electroretinogram (ERG):

a. the a-wave has negative deflection

b. a wave is generated by the retinal pigment epithelium

c. amacrine cells are responsible for the oscillatory potential

d. it is possible to separate the cone and rod ERG

Answer: a,c,d

353. With regard to pattern electroretinogram:

a. it can be used to estimate the visual acuity

b. it is generated by the occipital cortex

c. it is reduced in optic nerve diseases

d. the signal amplitude is about 10 mV

Answer: a, c,

354. The intraocular pressure:

a. shows a higher diurnal variation in glaucoma patients

b. is highest in the morning

c. gives a falsely higher reading in patients with thick cornea

d. all

Answer: d

355. The following are true about the cornea:

a. the stroma contains collagen fibrils of regular thickness

b. the Bowman's layer contains randomly arranged collagen fibrils

c. the Bowman's layer is the basement layer of the epithelium

d. type I collagen is the main type of collagen found in the cornea

Answer: a, b, d

356. Bleeding time is increased in:

a. massive blood transfusion

b. vitamin K deficiency

c. von Willebrand's disease
d. disseminated intravascular coagulation (DIC)

Answer: a, c, d

357. A shift in the oxygen-haemoglobin dissociation curve to the right occurs in :

a. hypothermia
b. carboxyhaemoglobin
c. acidosis
d. fetal haemoglobin

Answer: c

358. With regard to blood groups and blood products:

a. the ABO system is inherited in an autosomal dominant pattern
b. group O and Rhesus positive is the universal donors' blood.
c. stored whole blood contains dextrose, phosphate and citrate
d. stored blood becomes progressively more acidotic and hyperkalaemic with time

Answer: a, c, d

359. The following are true about platelets:

a. they are formed in the bone marrow from megakaryocytes.
b. their life span in circulation is about 30 days
c. in a normal person, 20% of the platelets are found in the spleen.
d. they contain adenosine diphophate and serotonin.

Answer: a, c, d

360. Haemoglobin SC disease:

a. is common amongst Afro-carribean people
b. does not show sickle cells in the blood film.
c. causes severe anaemia
d. causes retinal vein occlusion

Answer: a, d

361. The following are true about cardiac contraction:
a. the P wave initiates the atrial contraction

b. atrial contribution to ventricular filling is most effective at fast heart rate.

c. b wave is generated by atrial contraction

d. fourth heart sound occurs during atrial contraction

Answer: a, b, d

362. True statements about ECG include:

a. the P-R interval corresponds to the duration of atrial systole

b. the T-wave ends at the time of aortic valve closure

c. the ST segment represents repolarization of the ventricles

d. all

Answer: d

363. The following are true about micro-circulation:

a. arterioles have no muscle

b. capillaries have walls made up of a single layer of cells

c. capillaries have no innervation

d. the capillaries contain 5% of the total blood volume at any one time

Answer: b, c, d

364. Differences between myocardial muscles and normal muscles in that myocardial muscles:

a. can incur a greater oxygen debt

b. can metabolize lactic acid

c. contains no striated muscles

d. contains no glycogen

Answer: b

365. Oxygen blood supply to the heart depends on:

a. blood acidity

b. sympathetic tone

c. blood viscosity

d. all

Answer: d

366. The effect of noradrenaline on the heart include:
a. tachycardiac

b. increased duration of the cardiac action potential

c. decreased potassium conductance of the membranes of pacemaker cells

d. increased strength of cardiac contraction

Answer: a, d

367. The following are true about potassium:

a. hypokalaemia decreases the time of cardiac
   repolarization

b. hyperkalaemia decreases cardiac contraction

c. hyperkalaemia relaxes vascular smooth muscle

d. all

Answer: d

368. The following are true about aldosterone:

a. it is secreted by the adrenal medulla

b. its secretion is stimulated by decreased blood volume

c. it stimulates active reabsorption of sodium in the distal renal tubules.

d. it causes increased secretion of potassium by the distal renal tubules.

Answer: b, c, d

369. True statements about aldosterone include:

a. secretion is mainly under the control of adrenocorticotrophic (ACTH) hormone secretion

b. increases hepatic gluconeogenesis

c. its secretion is stimulated by angiotensin

d. in the kidney, mainly acts on the proximal convoluted tubules

Answer: c,

370. Following a major operation in a normal person, the following are seen:

a. fluid retention

b. decreased metabolic rate

c. potassium retention

d. decreased heart rate

Answer: a, b

371. The thyroid gland:
a. secretes clacitonin

b. arises from the base of the pharynx

c. contains about 100,000 follicles

d. has follicles lines a single layer of cells

Answer: a, b, d

372. The following are true:

a. thyroxine is formed by iodination of tyrosine

b. the ratio of T3 :T4 secreted by the thyroid gland is 1:5

c. about 99.5% of thyroxines is protein bound

d. T3 is more active than T4

Answer: a, c, d

373. The following are true about the hormones secreted by the adrenal cortex:

a. zona fasciculata secretes cortisol

b. zona glomerulosa secretes aldosterone

c. secretion of aldosterone is stimulated by ACTH

d. all

Answer: d

374. The following are true about calcium regulating hormones:

a. calcitonin increases the plasma calcium concentration

b. vitamin D is produced in the skin

c. vitamin D is metabolized to its active form in the liver and kidney.

d. vitamin D increases calcium absorption from the gut

Answer: b, c, d

375. Melatonin:

a. is secreted by pineal gland

b. regulates the circadian rhythm

c. is useful to regulate the sleep pattern of patients with complete blindness.

d. all

Answer: d

376. The following occur in untreated insulin dependent diabetes mellitus:
a. diuresis

b. decreased plasma amino acid

c. increased plasma fatty acid

d. ketonuria

Answer: a, c, d

377. Glucocorticoid causes an increase of:

a. red blood cells

b. lymphocytes

c. eosinophils

d. platelets

Answer: a, d

378. Angiotensin II:

a. is an octapeptide

b. is produced mainly in the lungs

c. causes thirst

d. all

Answer: d

379. Carbon dioxide in blood:

a. is more soluble than oxygen

b. is carried in combination with plasma

c. carries mainly as bicarbonate ions

d. all

Answer: d

380. In the human kidney:

a. renal plasma flow is normally 660 ml/minute

b. blood flow in the cortex is greater than that in the medulla

c. resorption of ions and water occurs mainly in the distal convoluted tubules

d. anti-diuretic hormone increases water resorption mainly in the distal convoluted tubules

Answer: a, b

381. The following reflexes are used to test brain stem death:
a. Babinski's reflexes

b. accommodation

c. gag reflex

d. vestibular-ocular reflex

Answer: c,d

382. The following are true about blood-brain barrier:

a. it is permeable at birth

b. it involves tight junction between endothelial cells and end feet processes of astrocytes

c. it is absent in the posterior pituitary

d. all above

Answer: d

383. True statements about cerebral blood flow:

a. it is controlled mainly by the autonomic nervous system

b. cerebral arterioles constricts when the blood pressure is raised

c. it is constant in the blood pressure range of 50 to 150 mm Hg systolic

d. hypocapnia increases the cerebral blood flow

Answer: b,c

384. Cerebrospinal fluid:

a. is produced mainly by the lateral, third and fourth ventricles

b. enters the subarachnoid space through foramina Lushka and Magendie

c. is reabsorbed mainly into the lymphatics

d. production is dependent of the blood pressure

Answer: a, b

385. Right abducent nerve palsy:

a. causes diplopia worse for distance than near

b. causes diplopia worse on right than left gaze

c. causes overaction of the left medial rectus

d. all above

Answer: d

386. With regard to cerebral blood flow:
a. is dependent on the intracranial pressure

b. is increased by hypoxia

c. is reduced by hypercapnia

d. is increased by hypothermia

Answer: a, b

387. In the heart:
a. excitation begins in the sinoatrial node

b. excitation of the ventricle begins at the apex and spread to the base

c. depolarization occurs from epicardium to endocardium

d. all above

Answer: d

388. Following acute haemorrhage, the following compensatory mechanisms occur:
a. increased chemoreceptor discharge

b. increased level of circulating angiotensin II

c. vasoconstriction of renal efferent arterioles

d. all above

Answer: d

389. With regard to insulin:
a. it is a 51 amino acid peptide

b. it is formed by removal of C-chain from proinsulin

c. it is produced by the alpha cells of the pancreas

d. it alters the rate of enzyme synthesis

Answer: a,b,d

390. The following are true about renal circulation:

a. it accounts for 25% of the cardiac output

b. it is regulated predominantly by the autonomic nervous system

c. in a normal 70 kg man, renal blood flow is about 1200ml/min

d. macula densa cells are found in the efferent arteriolar wall

Answer: a,c,d

391. With regard to the choroid:
a. the choroid receives 85% of blood flow to the eye

b. the blood vessels in the choroid contains tight junction

c. the choroid vessels are embedded in a matrix made up of type III collagen

d. in the presence of high partial pressure of carbon dioxide the choroidal vessels increase in diameter

Answer: a,c,d

392. True statements about the pupil include:

a. it is controlled mainly by the autonomic system

b. miosis increases the depth of focus for near vision

c. a change in the pupil diameter from 2 to 8 mm increases the amount of light entering the eye by 16-fold

d. all above

Answer: d

393. The following are true about iris:
a. it receives 5% of total blood flow

b. it contains blood vessels with radial coils

c. it contains fenestration in the blood vessels

d. the sympathetic activity in the iris dilator muscles
   is mainly mediated by □ receptors

Answer: a,b

394. True statements about the retinal blood flow include:
a. the retina receives 5% of total ocular blood flow

b. the retinal blood flow is mainly under the sympathetic
   control

c. the retina blood vessels are impermeable to ascorbate

d. the pericytes control the contractile activity of the retinal
   blood vessels

Answer: a, d

395. The following are true about the aqueous:

a. the protein content of aqueous is about 1/5 that of the plasma

b. the main type of protein found in the aqueous is transferrin

c. Ig G is found in the aqueous

d. stimulation of □2 receptors reduces aqueous production

Answer: c, d

396. Thyroid hormone:
a. increases the absorption of carbohydrate from the intestine

b. exerts a negative feedback action on TSH production

c. increases the concentration of 2,3-DPG within the red blood cells

d. all above

Answer: d

397. Aldosterone:
a. increases mRNA synthesis

b. deficiency results in hypotension

c. increases sodium reabsorption from sweat

d. all above

Answer: d

398. Insulin:
a. has a half-lilfe of 60 minutes

b. stimulate glycolysis in liver and muscle

c. stimulate lipogenesis in liver and fat tissues

d. is synthesized in the endoplasmic reticulum of the□ beta cells

Answer: c, d

399. Calcitonin:
a. is a steroid hormone

b. is produced by the parafollicular cells within the thyroid glands

c. is increased in the presence of hypercalcaemia

d. inhibits osteoclast activity

Answer: b, c, d

400. Parathyroid hormone:

a. is a peptide hormone

b. is released in response to hypocalcaemia

c. increases phosphate reabsorption in the kidneys

d. increases calcium excretion in the kidneys

Answer: a, b

401. The following are true about an action potential in a nerve fibre:
a. it occurs when its membrane potential is hyperpolarized

b. it is associated with a transient increase in membrane permeability to sodium

c. there is a decreased in membrane permeability to potassium

d. it has an amplitude which varies directly to the strength of stimulus

Answer: b, c

402. Increased intracranial pressure causes:
a. sixth nerve palsy

b. cupping of the optic disc

c. absent venous pulsation

d. increased cerebral blood flow

Answer: a, c

403. Muscle tone is reduced by:
a. lower motor neurone lesion

b. curare

c. cerebellar lesion

d. all above

Answer: d

404. Optic disc swelling occurs in:
a. optic disc drusen

b. hypotony

c. central retinal vein occlusion

d. retrobulbar neuritis

Answer: b, c

405. Compared with myelinated nerve fibres, non-myelinated nerve fibres :

a. have a higher threshold for stimulation

b. have a longer refractory period

c. transmit impulses at a lower frequency

d. all above

Answer: d

406. The following are neurotransmitters at the autonomic post-ganglionic nerve endings:
a. GABA

b. noradrenaline

c. acetylcholine

d. 5 HT

Answer: b, c

407. The following are neurotransmitters in the autonomic ganglia:
a. GABA

b. noradrenaline

c. acetylcholine

d. 5 HT

Answer: c

408. An increase in $PaCO_2$ lead to:

a. hypertension

b. increased adrenaline release

c. increased sweating

d. all above

Answer: d

409. Stimulation of the beta receptors give rise to:

a. tachycardia

b. increased myocardial contraction

c. vasoconstriction of visceral vessels

d. pupil dilatation

Answer: a,b

410. Valsalva manoeuvre causes:

a. increased peripheral resistance

b. raised in intraocular pressure

c. drop in blood pressure

c

411. Pupil dilatation occurs with:
a. neostigmine

b. cocaine

c. atenolol

d. codeine

Answer: b

412. Vitamin B12 deficiency causes:

a. optic atrophy

b. papilloedema

c. centrocecal scotoma

d. loss of position sense

Answer: c, d

413. The effect of glucagon include:

a. ketogenesis

b. glycogenolysis

c. gluconeogenesis

d. all above

Answer: d

414. Cytochrome P450 is:

a. involves in phase I metabolic reactions

b. found in lysosomes

c. found in hepatocytes

d. found in mitochondria

Answer: a, c

415. Balance salt solution (BSS) used in cataract surgery contains:

a. mannitol

b. calcium chloride

c. magnesium chloride

d. acetate

Answer: b, c, d

416. Vasodilators produced by the endothelium include:
a. endothelium derived relaxing factor (EDRF)

b. nitric oxide (NO)

c. prostacyclin (PGL2)

d. all above

Answer: d

417. Actions of angiotensin II include:

a. increases the release of aldosterone

b. reduces renin release from the kidney

c. vasodilatation

d. promotes microalbuminuria

Answer: a, b, d

418. The following cranial nerves contain parasympathetic outflow arising at the brain stem:

a. optic nerve

b. oculomotor nerve

c. trigeminal nerve

d. facial nerve

Answer: b, d

419. In a normal nephron:

a. the descending loop of Henle is impermeable to water

b. anti-diuretic hormone (ADH) increases the permeability of collecting ducts to water

c. all the filtered glucose is re-absorbed in the proximal tubule

d. nearly all the filtered protein is reabsorbed in the proximal convoluted tubule

Answer: b, c, d

420. Sudden assumption of an upright position from supine position causes an initial decrease in::

a. cardiac output

b. heart rate

c. cerebral blood flow

d. total peripheral resistance

Answer: a, c

421. The release of neurotransmitter from synaptic vesicles:
a. takes place by exocytosis

b. is controlled by neuronal calcium influx

c. is quantal

d. all above

Answer: d

422. The following are true about acetylcholine:

a. it has a strong affinity for nicotinic receptors

b. is derived from acetyl CoA and choline

c. is synthesized by a reaction involving choline acetyltransferase

d. all above

Answer: d

423. The effect of calcium ions on neurotransmitter release at synapses include:

a. vesicular fusion

b. tonic depolarization of the presynaptic neurone

c. post-tetanic potentiation

d. all above

Answer: d

424. The neuronal resting membrane of the human brain is :

a. maintained by the sodium pump

b. around -70mV

c. maintained by using ATP for energy

d. all above

Answer: d

425. In rapid eye movement sleep, the following are seen:
a. increased heart rate

b. increased systolic blood pressure

c. decreased respiratory rate

d. all above

Answer: a, b

426. The following are true about the lens:
a. it has a higher concentration of sodium than potassium

b. it has the highest concentration of protein than other organs in the body

c. 90% of proteins in the lens are water-soluble

d. gluthatione is reduced in cataract

Answer: b, c, d

427. The felderstrukter fibres of the extraocular muscles:

a. form the bulk of the orbital part of the muscle

b. have poorly developed sarcoplasmic reticulum

c. are singly innervated

d. are more richly supplied by blood than the fibrillenstrukter fibres

Answer: b,

428. The following are true about rods in darkness:

a. there is tonic release of neurotransmitters

b. the sodium ion channels are open

c. the potassium ion channels are shut

d. there is a net influx of sodium ions

Answer: a, b, d

429. When a photon strikes the rhodopsin:

a. bleaching occurs

b. retinal molecules are bound to rhodopsin

c. the intracellular cGMP is increased

d. the sodium ion channels are closed

Answer: a, d

430. A lesion in the right medial longitudinal fasciculus:
a. causes left abduction nystagmus

b. impairs right adduction

c. impairs left adduction

d. causes problem with upgaze

Answer: a, b

431. Inhibition of the Edinger-Westphal nucleus:
a. causes relaxation of the iris sphincter

b. causes contraction of the iris dilator

c. occurs in deep sleep

d. occurs with narcotics

Answer: a, b

432. The following are involved in colour vision:
a. P pathway

b. M pathway

c. area V8 of visual cortex

d. area V3 of visual cortex

Answer: a, c

433. The following are true about saccade:
a. it has a higher velocity than pursuit movements

b. the visual acuity is increased during saccades

c. horizontal saccade is controlled by the pons

d. vertical saccade is controlled by the mid-brain

Answer: a, c, d

434. True statements about visual adaptation include:
a. light adaptation takes longer than dark adaptation

b. dark adaptation reaches its maximum in about 20 minutes

c. in dark adapted eye, a higher intensity of light is required to stimulate cones than rods

d. people who wear red goggles in the light adapt quicker in the dark than those who do not wear them

Answer: b, c

435. With regard to light perception:
a. the fovea contains only cones

b. the cones have a lower threshold to light than rods

c. rods respond most to the red-yellow end of light

d. rods respond most to wavelengths of about 500nm

Answer: a, d

436. Urine volume is increased with:
a. carbonic anhydrase inhibitors

b. hyperglycaemia

c. increased aldosterone secretion

d. damage to the posterior pituitary

Answer: a, b, d

437. With regard to the transport of carbon dioxide in blood:

a. 25% of carbon dioxide is dissolved in blood

b. carbonic anhydrase is found in plasma

c. 50% of carbon dioxide is carried as bicarbonate

d. deoxygenated haemoglobin facilitates the transport of carbon dioxide

Answer: d

438. The following are true about cerebrospinal fluid:
a. it has a greater buffering capacity than plasma

b. it has a similar chloride concentration to plasma

c. it is a plasma ultrafiltrate

d. the rate of formation is dependent on the intraventricular pressure over the normal pressure range

Answer: c

439. True statements about the pH of the extracellular fluid:
a. in healthy people it is maintained between 7.4 and 7.5

b. is increased in hypovolaemic shock

c. decreases following a cardiac arrest

d. influences the binding of drugs to plasma proteins

Answer: c, d

440. The following occur in the proximal tubules of the nephron:
a. reabsorption of all glucose

b. reabsorption of most water

c. secretion of bicarbonate

d. active reabsorption of sodium

Answer: a, b, d

441. The effect of stellate ganglion block include:
a. anhydrosis

b. dilated conjunctival vessels

c. ptosis

d. all above

Answer: d

442. Parasympathetic ganglia include:
a. Gasserian ganglion

b. otic ganglion

c. stellate ganglion

d. celiac ganglion

Answer: b

443. With regard to knee jerk:
a. it is a monosynaptic reflex

b. the impulse travels via type Ia afferent fibres

c. the Golgi body is an important component

d. the stimulus begins in the tendon

Answer: a, b

444. In myasthenia gravis:
a. the vertical muscles of the eye are more commonly involved than the horizontal muscles

b. the pupil reaction to light is sluggish

c. absent antibody to acetylcholine receptors exclude the diagnosis

d. Cogan's twitch refers to involuntary twitching of the orbicularis

Answer: a

445. Relative afferent pupillary defect is seen in:
a. age-related macular degeneration

b. optic nerve glioma

c. unilateral occipital lobe infarction

d. third nerve palsy

Answer: b

446. The following are true about the sensitivity of the visual system:
a. in the dark the peak sensitivity of the eye is around 500nm

b. in the light the peak sensitivity of the eye is around 555nm

c. the cone can not respond to white flickering light of 20 Hz and above

d. a dark-adapted eye is more sensitive to blue-green light than a light-adapted eye

Answer: a,b,d

447. Purkinje's shift:
a. refers to the transition of retinal sensitivity between photopic and scotopic vision

b. refers to the shift in the spectral sensitivity of the human retina toward shorter wavelengths of light

c. accounts for blue colour appearing brighter at dusk

d. all above

Answer: d

448. In a patient with dense cataract and poor retina view, the following tests can be used to test the macular function:
a. relative afferent pupillary defect

b. laser interferometry

c. Haidinger brushes

d. Visual evoked potential

Answer: b, c, d

449. The release of acetylcholine is blocked by:

a. hemicholinum

b. venom of black widow spider

c. cocaine

d. botulinum toxins

Answer: b, d

450. The following are true:
a. Kirschman's law: the greatest contrast in colour is seen when the luminosity differnece is small

b. Emmbert's law: the perceived size of an object varies in proportion to the distance of the surface on which it is projected

c. Hering's law: the contraction of a muscle is accompanied by simultaneous and proportional relaxation of the antagonist

d. Troxler's phenomenon: an image in the periphery of the retina tends to fade or disappear during steady fixation of another object

Answer: a, b, d

451. Antidiuretic hormone:

a. decreases the osmolarity of urine

b. decreases the volume of urine

c. increases the reabsorption of water in the proximal tubules

d. is synthesized in the posterior pituitary gland

Answer: b

452. Insulin secretion:
a. is inhibited by atropine

b. is increased by vagal stimulation

c. is inhibited by amino acids

d. is stimulated by beta agonists

Answer: a, b

453. Prolactin secretion:
a. is higher in female than male

b. is inhibited by dopamine

c. is increased in patients taking phenothiazines

d. all above

Answer: d.

454. Melatonin:
a. is secreted by pineal body

b. secretion is highest at night

c. secretion is inhibited by light

d. all above

Answer: d.

455. Cortisol:

a. increases the circulating lymphocytes

b. increases the circulating eosinophils

c. decreases the production of prostaglandins

d. inhibits the production of fibroblasts

Answer: a, c, d

456. Vasodilatation occurs in:
a. increased lactate concentration.
b. decreased in skin temperature

c. increased hydrogen ions concentration

d. increased in potassium concentration

Answer: a, c, d

457. The effects of stress include:

a. increased testosterone secretion

b. decreased insulin secretion

c. increased prolactin secretion

d. increased ADH secretion

Answer: b, c, d

458. Hyperventilation:
a. decreases cerebral blood flow

b. increases ionized calcium concentration in the serum

c. causes hypocapnia

d. causes metabolic alkalosis

Answer: a, c,

459. Pain from local anaesthesia injection can be reduced by:
a. warming the local anaesthetic

b. quick injection

c. using a needle with a small bore

d. adding sodium bicarbonate in the local anaesthetic

Answer: a, c, d

460. The following solutions are isotonic (same osmolarity as the plasma):

a. Harman's solution

b. 0.9% saline

c. 10% mannitol

d. 5% glucose

 Answer: a, b, d

461. Regarding the kidneys:
a. there are 1.3 millions nephrons in each kidney
b. they produce the aldosterone

c. they receive 12% of the cardiac output when at rest

d. they produce 1.25-dihydroxycalciferol

Answer: a, d

462. Aldosterone secretion is controlled by:

a. plasma sodium concentration

b. plasma calcium concentration

c. plasma potassium concentration

d. angiotensin II

Answer: a, c, d

463. In pregnancy:
a. the lysozyme in the tear film is increased

b. the intraocular pressure is lower than pre-pregnancy state

c. accommodation is decreased

d. all above

Answer: d

464. The following findings are normal in pregnancy:
a. elevated erythrocyte sedimentation rate (ESR)

b. raised serum urea

c. raised serum creatinine

d. elevated white blood cell count

Answer: a, d

465. With regard to cerebral autoregulation:

a. cerebral blood flow is constant over a diastolic blood pressure of 60 to 140 mmHg

b. autoregulation is lost during the acute phase of subarachnoid haemorrhage

c. it is impaired in hypercapnia

d. it is impaired in hypoxia

Answer: b, c, d

466. The following are true about critical fusion frequency:
a. it refers to the rate at which stimuli can be presented and still be perceived as separate stimuli
b. it is dependent on visual acuity

c. it is dependent on the spacing between neighbouring photoreceptors

d. it depends on the time-resolving ability of the eye

Answer: a, d

467. Structures involved in colour vision include:

a. parvocellular pathway

b. superficial layer 4C of visual cortex

c. superior collliculi

d. geniculate layers 1-2

Answer: a,

468. Area(s) in the visual cortex involved in colour vision include:
a. V1

b. V2

c. V3

d. V8

Answer: d

469. Differences between the M cells and P cells include:
a. M cells have larger cell bodies than P cells

b. M cells have slower conduction rate than P cells

c. M cells have larger receptive field than P cells

d. M cells do not synapse in lateral geniculate body whereas P cells do

Answer: a, c

470. The superior colliculi:

a. receives P fibres from the retina

b. receives M fibres from the retina

c. regulates saccade movement

d. is the centre for pursuit movement

Answer: b, c

471. The Bell's phenomenon:
a. occurs during normal blinking

b. if absent suggests brain stem disease

c. is absent in Bell's palsy

d. is reduced or absent in patients with thyroid orbitopathy

Answer: d

472. The following are true about pupil reaction to light:

a. secretion of acetylcholine is responsible for pupil dilatation

b. constriction of the pupil is mediated by nerve fibres travelling in the short ciliary nerve

c. dilatation of the pupil is mediated by nerve fibres travelling in the long ciliary nerve

d. the sympathetic nerve innervates the dilator muscles

Answer: b, c, d

473. a. it receives input from the semi-circular canal

b. it receives input from the otolith

c. it is suppressed when the object is moving with the subject

d. all above

Answer: d

474. The human lens:
a. is innervated by the ophthalmic nerve

b. has a uniform refractive index

c. has a large radius of curvature anteriorly than posteriorly

d. stops growing after birth

Answer: c

475. The following are true about the ERG:

a. in infarction of the choroidal circulation the a-wave of the ERG is reduced or absent

b. the ERG is always abnormal in patients with macular diseases

c. flicker ERG can be used to isolate cone photoreceptors

d. the b-wave of ERG is reduced in dark-adapted eye

Answer: a, c, d

476. The bright-flash ERG:
a. comes only from the cones

b. is generated in a fully dark adapted eye by the highest intensity of light

c. can be used to assess the overall retinal integrity in the presence of media opacity

d. is abnormal in patients with age-related macular degeneration

Answer: b, c,

477. The following cells contribute the wavefronts of the flash ERG:

a. retinal pigment epithelium

b. corneal endothelium

c. photoreceptors

d. ganglion cells

Answer: a, c,

478. The parameters that are measured clinically in the flash ERG are:

a. amplitude

b. excitation time

c. implicit time

d. latency

Answer: a, c,

479. The following methods can be used to test solely the rod ERG:
a. a rapidly flickering light

b. red light stimulus

c. low-density blue light in dark adapted eye

d. focal ERG

Answer: c

480. Pattern ERG (PERG):

a. tests the function of the ganglion cells

b. uses a checkeredboard pattern that changes in luminance

c. gives the same information as visual evoked response (VER)

d. is abnormal in glaucoma

Answer: a, c, d

481. With regard to nystagmus:
a. caloric nystagmus occurs when iced water is poured into the ear

b. vestibular nystagmus occurs as a consequence of head rotation

c. optokinetic nystagmus occurs as a consequence of the relative motion of the visual field

d. all above

Answer: d

482. Visual-evoked response:

a. is used primarily to detect visual loss due to retinal disease

b. produces biphasic wavefronts

c. may give falsely delayed latency if the patient is not concentrating

d. produces responses in normal subjects with a latency of 100msec

Answer: c, d

483. An increase in intra-ocular pressure occurs with:

a. normal blinking

b. coughing

c. hypercarbia

d. all above

Answer: d

484. With regard to dark adaptation:
a. is a quicker process than light adaptation

b. the sensitivity of the cones increases more rapidly than the rods

c. it is monophasic in rod monochromatism

d. the first limb of the curve represents rod recovery

Answer: b, c

485. True statements about EOG (electro-oculogram) include:

a. the EOG light-peak to dark-trough ratio is reduced in central retinal vein occlusion

b. the light peak of EOG is abnormal in Best's disease

c. the EOG light rise is produced by depolarization of the basal membrane of the retinal pigment epithelium

d. all above

Answer: d

486. The following may cause an elevated blood urea:
a. renal disease

b. steroid therapy

c. dehydration

d. all above

Answer: d

487. The following occur in response to a major surgery:

a. increased potassium loss

b. increased protein breakdown

c. sodium and water retention

d. all above

Answer: d

488. Hyperventilation causes:

a. an alkaline urine

b. a fall in the plasma bicarbonate concentration

c. increased cardiac output

d. all above

Answer: d

489. Bradycardiac can occur in response to:
a. elevated intraocular pressure

b. ocular massage

c. pulling of the extraocular muscle

d. all above

Answer: d

490. The following are true about the Troxler's phenomenon:

a. it refers to disappearance of an image during steady fixation of another object

b. it only occurs in the peripheral retina

c. eye movement eliminates this phenomenon

d. movement of the object eliminates this phenomenon

Answer: a, c, d

491. The following are true:
a. a horopter is a straight line on which an object will stimulate corresponding retinal points

b. objects further or nearer than the horopter to the eyes are always perceived as double

c. objects in the Panum's area are perceived singly

d. objects outside the Panum's are are perceived as double

Answer: c, d

492. Doll's head phenomenon:

a. refers to movement of the eyes in a direction opposite to which the head is suddenly moved

b. elicits both horizontal and vertical vestibuloocular reflexes

c. is absent in patients with brain stem death

d. all above

Answer: d

493. The following are true about ocular circulation:
a. only 4% of the total blood supply to the eye goes to the retina

b. the choroidal blood flow in normal people is ten times that of the grey mater of the brain

c. autoregulation occurs in both retinal and choroidal circulation

d. a PaCO2 rise of 1 mm Hg induces a 3% rise in retinal blood flow

Answer: a, b, d

494. The following may explain why a patient who had had a relative afferent pupillary defect has normal pupillary reaction to light:
a. removal of a cataract

b. resolution of optic neuritis

c. anterior ischaemic optic neuropathy in both eyes

d. development of bilateral papilloedema

Answer: b, c

495. In efferent pupillary defect:

a. anisocoria is present

b. the damage may be in the visual cortex

c. the damage may be in the superior colliculus

d. all above

Answer: d

496. With regard to efferent pupillary defect:
a. the pupil reacts poorly to light and accommodation

b. anisocoria is a feature

c. the affected eye has poor distant vision

d. a lesion in the sympathetic pathway is a recognized
   cause

Answer: a, b, d

497. The following are true about corneal sensation:
a. the sensation is greatest at the apex and diminishes towards the limbus.

b. the temporal half of the cornea is more sensitive than the nasal half

c. the Bonnet-Cochet aesthesiometer gives quantitative measure of the degree of hypoaesthesia

d. all above

Answer: d

498. The following are true about spectral sensitivity of the retina:
a. in scotopic conditions, the peak sensitivity of the eye is near 500 nm

b. under photopic conditions the peak sensitivity is near 555 nm

c. in the presence of a bright yellow steady background light the retina has a peak sensitivity near 440 nm to a 25-Hz stimulus

d. all above

Answer: d

499. Regarding retinal metabolism:
a. insulin is essential for the uptake of glucose by the retina

b. anaerobic metabolism predominates

c. the pigment retinal epithelium stores glycogen and supplies the need of the retina

d. the demand of oxygen is met entirely by the central retinal artery

Answer: b

500. The following conditions are required for rhodopsin regeneration:
a. NADPH

b. darkness

c. splitting of all trans-retinal from the opsin

d. all above

Answer: d